"For You created my inmost being; You knit me together in my mother's womb. I praise You because I am fearfully and wonderfully made; Your works are wonderful, I know that full well."

Psalm 139:13-14

Being a mother is the greatest blessing a woman is ever given. Pregnancy can be very difficult, sometimes even the most difficult of things, but the rewards that come from it literally last a lifetime. Congratulations!

Jessica & The Girls

3/2007

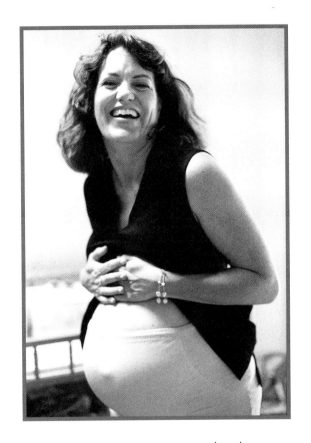

waiting for my baby

waiting for my

Baby

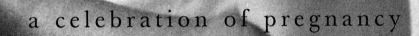

a celebration of pregnancy

Edited by Linda Sunshine

Designed by Pat Tan

STARK BOOKS

**Andrews McMeel
Publishing**

Kansas City

ATTENTION: SCHOOLS AND BUSINESSES
Andrews McMeel books are available at quantity discounts with
bulk purchase for educational, business, or sales promotional use.
For information, please write to:
Special Sales Department, Andrews McMeel Publishing,
4520 Main Street, Kansas City, Missouri 64111.

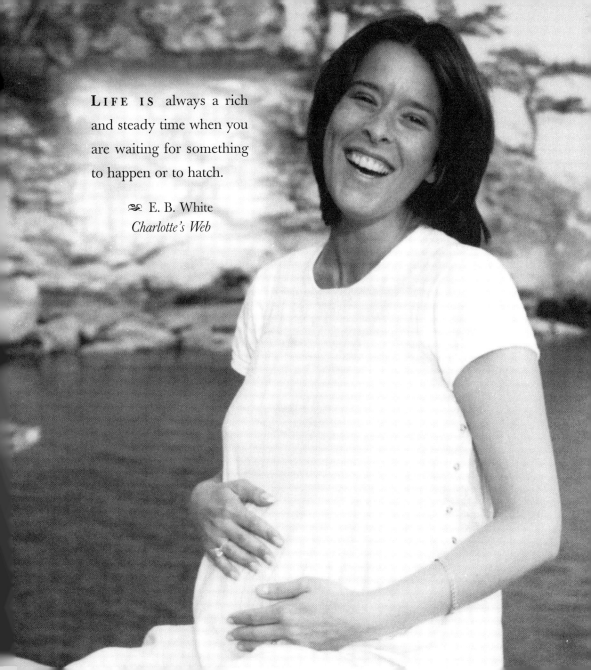

LIFE IS always a rich
and steady time when you
are waiting for something
to happen or to hatch.

❧ E. B. White
Charlotte's Web

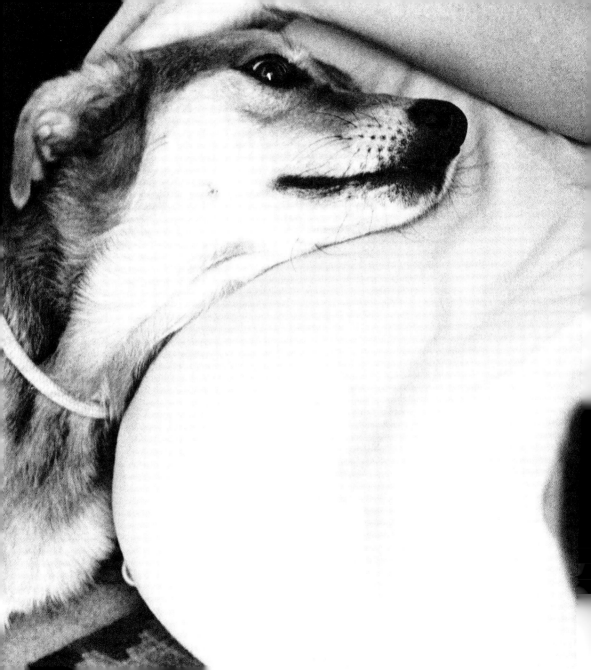

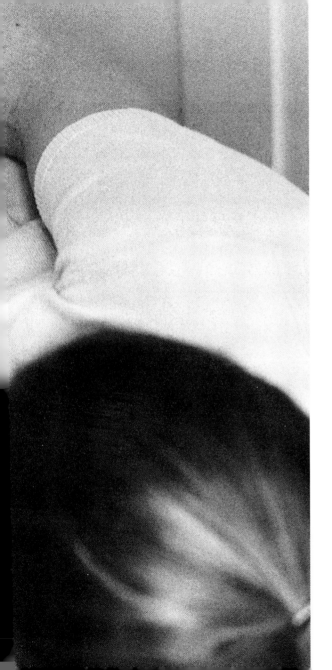

MAKING the decision to have a child ~ it's momentous. It is to decide forever to have your heart go walking around outside your body.

≈ Elizabeth Stone

OFTEN **I** AM FILLED WITH HOPE; sometimes I am consumed with dread. Often I feel blessed; sometimes I feel resentful. Sometimes I am downright giddy. Sometimes I'm so sentimental an AT&T commercial sends me over the edge. Sometimes I feel gorgeous, earthy and powerful. Sometimes I feel like a helium balloon with gravity shoes. . . .

A delusion, you say? Certainly not. Look, I'm not crazy ~ I'm pregnant.

ॐ Arlene Modica Matthews
Excited, Exhausted, Expecting

LIFE IS THE FIRST GIFT, love is the second and understanding the third.

ॐ Marge Piercy

EVERY MOTHER LIKES TO TELL YOU the story of their baby's birth. It's a bonding experience and no one can resist. Just don't pay too much attention to the awful ones. Instead, smile and nod your head. Pretty soon you'll have your own stories to frighten expectant mothers with.

> ❧ Ingrid Barth, as quoted in *On the Birth of Your Child* by Sherry Conway Appel

TO HEIR IS HUMAN.

> ❧ Marlene Cox, *Ladies' Home Journal*

ENVY THE KANGAROO. The pouch set-up is extraordinary; the baby crawls out of the womb when it is about two inches long, gets into the pouch and proceeds to mature. I'd have a baby if it would develop in my handbag.

> ❧ Rita Rudner, *Naked Beneath My Clothes*

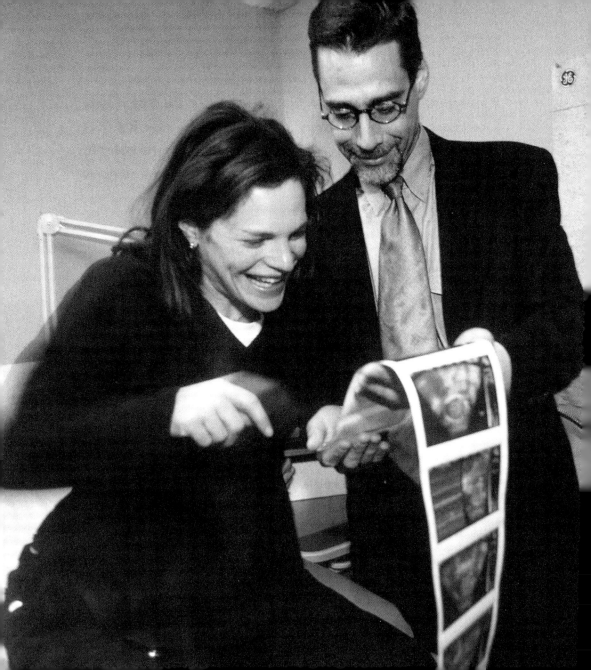

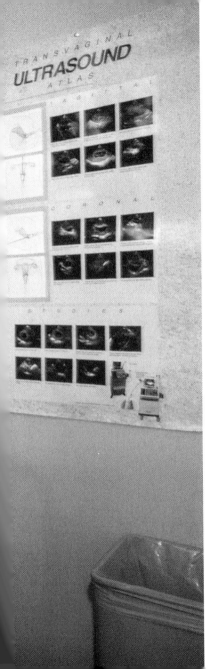

I CRIED WHEN THE ULTRASOUND technician told me the baby is a girl. How will I protect her? How will I accept that I can't? Each time I feel one of her kicks, already signaling her independence, I feel a blend of joy and wonder and fear and grief unlike anything I've known before.

❧ Hope Edelman, *The Mother Connection*

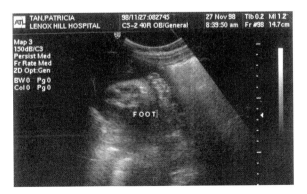

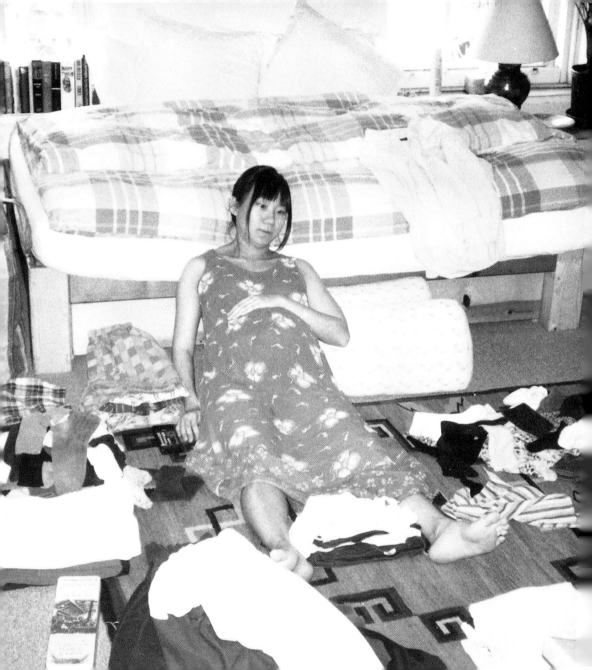

K NOWING THAT I AM PREGNANT makes me even more tired. Sometimes when I get home from work, I fall asleep on the couch before eating.

      ❧ Rachel A. Silverman, *Bastille*

E VERY PREGNANT WOMAN should be surrounded with every possible comfort.

      ❧ Dr. Flora L. S. Aldrich
      The Boudoir Companion

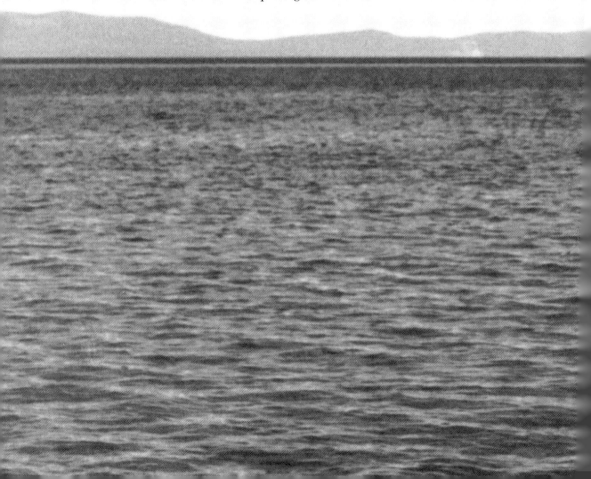

WHEN MY BABY WAS INSIDE ME, I felt his energy.
I knew he would be very intellectual, spiritual and methodic, and he is.

≈ Marcela Washington
Shape magazine

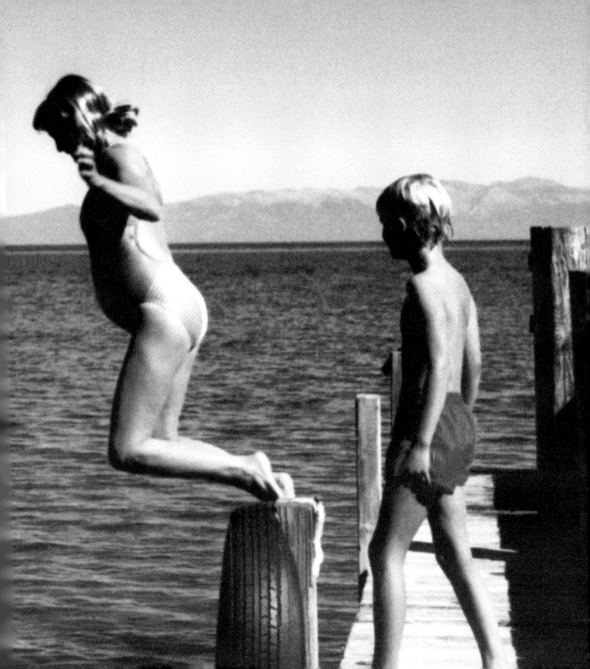

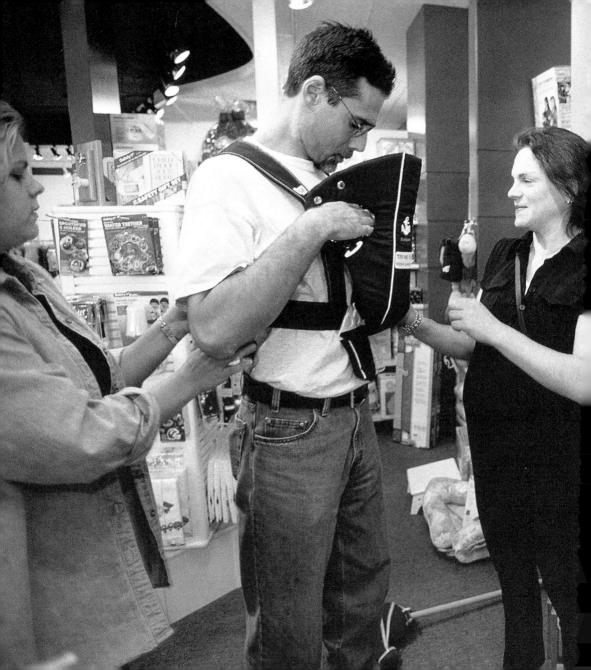

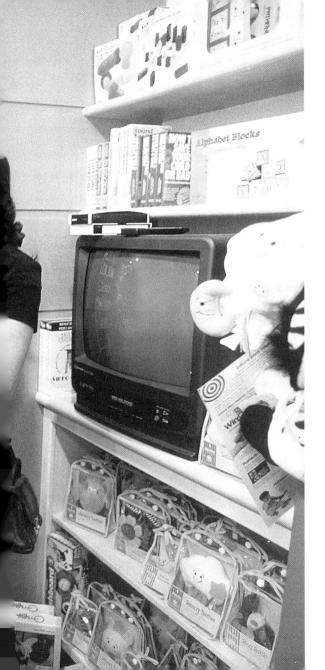

KEEPING a baby requires a great deal of time, effort, thought and equipment, so unless you are prepared for this, we recommend that you start with a hamster, whose wants are far simpler.

❧ Elinor Goulding Smith
*The Complete Book of Absolutely
Perfect Baby and Child Care*

S o I a m o f t e n a w a k e these days in the hours before dawn, full of joy, full of fear. The first birds begin to sing at quarter after five, and when Sam moves around in my stomach, kicking, it feels like there are trout inside me, leaping, and I go in and out of the aloneness, in and out of that sacred place.

❧ Annie Lamott
Some Thoughts on Being Pregnant

I f e e l s o b l e s s e d to be given the opportunity to host a new life. I go about my daily activities yet I am a universe unto myself, building bones, eyes, brain and heart. To be pregnant is to almost grasp the supernatural energy that surrounds our lives.

❧ L. J. Mark
Big Apple Parent

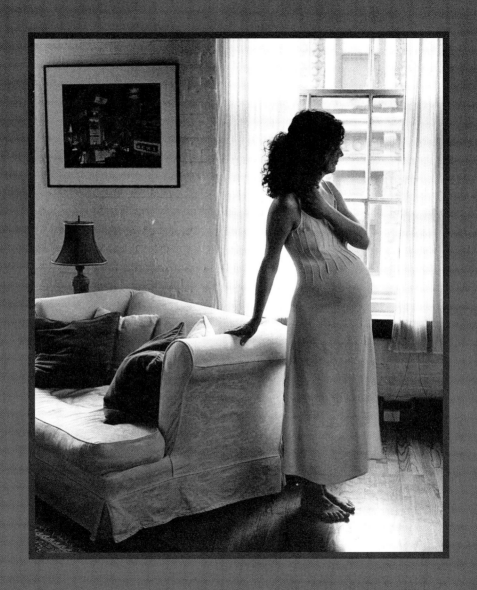

WOMEN ARE STRONG, strong, terribly strong. We don't know how strong we are until we're pushing out our babies.

❧ Louise Erdrich, *The Blue Jay's Dance*

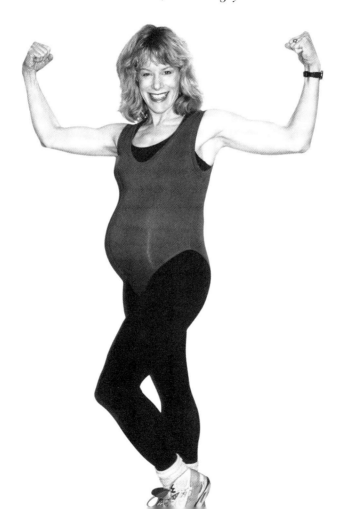

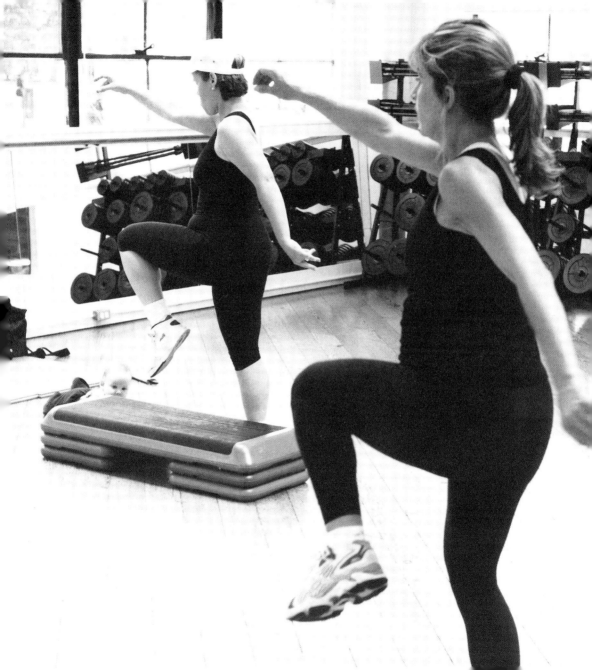

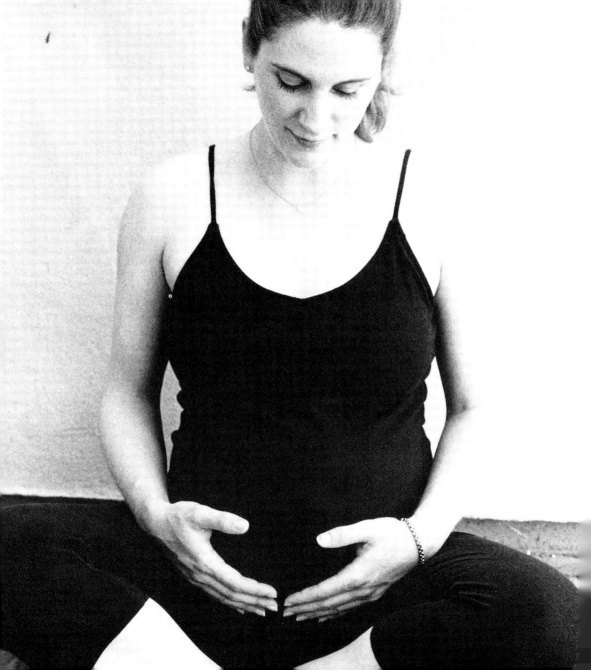

THIS IS MY FIRST PREGNANCY and it's been surprisingly easy and really fun. I am constantly laughing at myself and my belly. I'm always petting my baby and he really responds. When he comes out, he'll want to do yoga and have a daily massage.

≈ Amy Knudsen

I LOVE KNOWING there's this beautiful new being growing inside of me. I love hearing the heartbeat for the first time. I love when he responds to my voice and I feel him play inside me. . . . I love sharing the joy of pregnancy, talking about a safe, happy delivery. I love buying clothes and the little things my baby will need. I love knowing my body is participating in one of the greatest miracles. I love the way my body feels ~ fertile, pregnant and alive!

≈ Mary Liz Murphy
as quoted in *Fit Pregnancy* magazine

I AM CONFUSED BY EVERYTHING. . . . My big tummy is making the decisions now. The bigger it gets, the more I live in it. Me and my big tummy are the entire world and I don't care about anything else.

☙ Anne H. Mavor
Mother Tongue: A Performance Pregnancy Diary

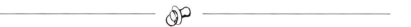

PREGNANCY is a total body experience. You must be shocked on a daily basis about how much control that little tyrant has over the rest of you. Your emotions, your complexion, your sex drive, your hair growth are all affected by the baby. This is when you must learn to surrender and realize that this child has you in its spell until the day you die.

☙ Vicki Iovine
The Girlfriend's Guide to Pregnancy Daily Diary

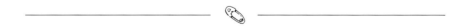

. . . ALL MY BODY IS A VEIL beneath which a child sleeps.

☙ Gabriela Mistral, "To My Husband"

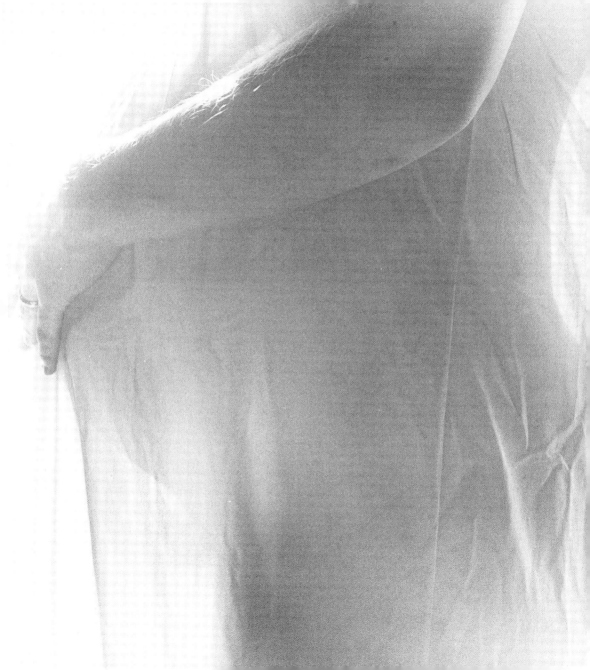

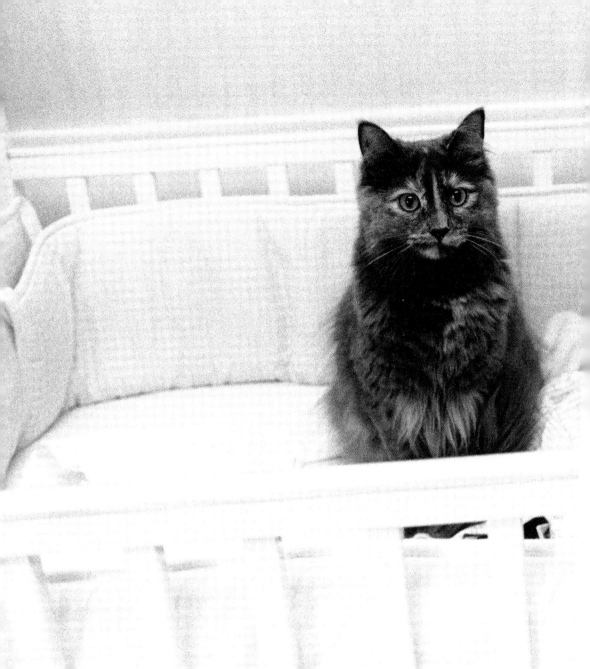

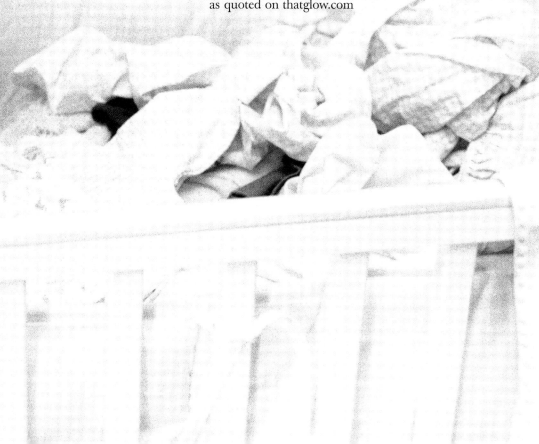

DURING MY PREGNANCY I was so hormonal, especially in the last three weeks. There's that song from *Dumbo,* "Baby of Mine," which the mother elephant sings to her baby from jail. Every time I would think of that song, I'd burst into tears.

≈ Reese Witherspoon
as quoted on thatglow.com

I BEGAN TO HAVE AN IDEA of my life, not as the slow shaping of achievement to fit my preconceived purposes, but as a gradual discovery and growth of purpose which I did not know.

❧ Joanna Field

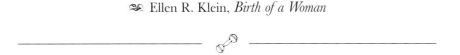

I AM IN AWE of the fact that within me lives a person who is the collective sum of all our ancestors. I am excited, elated and euphoric.

And unsettled.

❧ Ellen R. Klein, *Birth of a Woman*

I WANTED MY CHILD to grow up happy. And since life can be awkward, I wanted him or her to have enough good luck and good sense to keep happiness forever within reach. I hoped, too, that my child would always feel comfortable talking things over with me. Someday soon over apple juice and hot chocolate; sometime later over wine and coffee.

That's what I wanted. I wanted my child to be my friend. I wanted to pass the torch to a friend.

❧ Carol Weston, *From Here to Maternity*

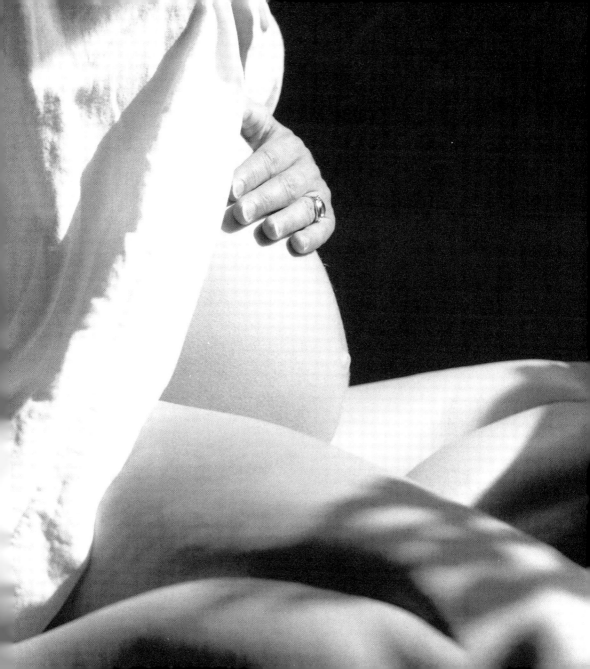

MOTHERHOOD IS A STORM, A SEIZURE: It is like weather. Nights of high wind, followed by calm mornings of brilliant sunshine that gives way to tropical rain, or blinding snow.

❧ Laurie Colwin, *A Big Storm Knocked It Over*

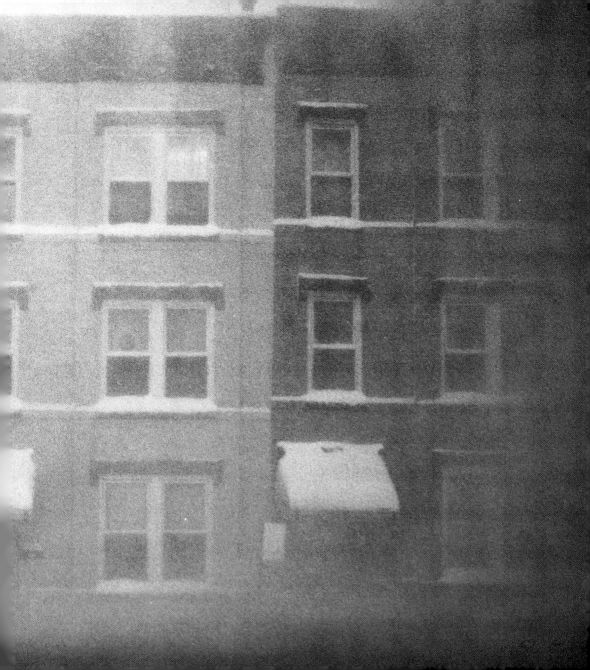

EVERY MOTHER contains her daughter in herself and every daughter her mother. Every woman extends backwards into her mother and forward into her daughter.

❧ Carl Jung

ONE MOTHER SAYS that she casually asked her two-year-old if she remembered being in the womb. Her daughter looked up at her, smiled and said, "Yup, I remember I used to tickle you with my feet."

❧ Dennis Brown, M.D., and Pamela Toussaint
*Mama's Little Baby: The Black Woman's Guide to Pregnancy,
Childbirth and Baby's First Year*

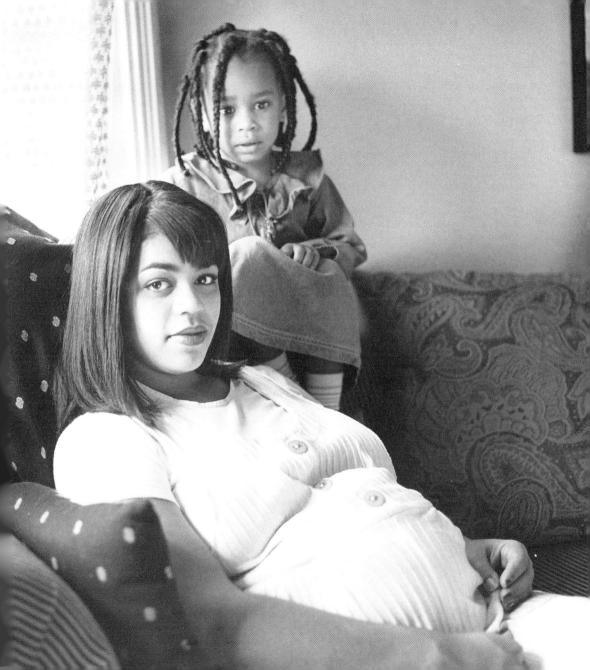

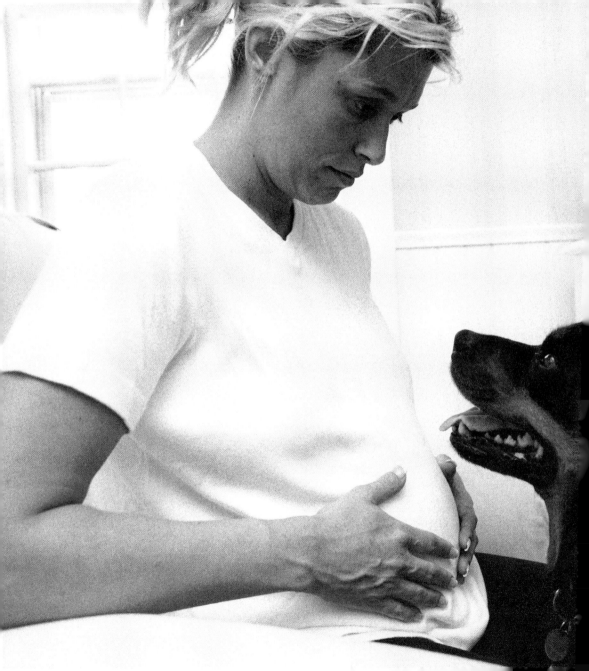

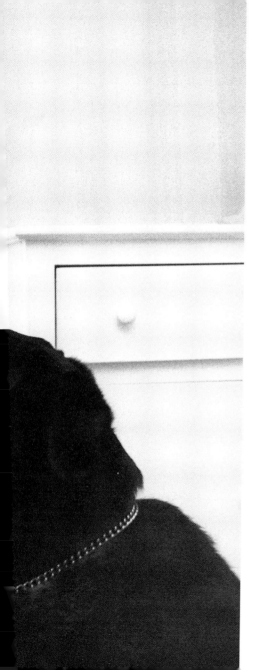

QUIT TURNING to someone else to do your thinking. You see that little squirrel out there in that tree? She has babies, and she has never read a book. Maybe it is not quite that simple, but it is not half as complicated as the books, neighbors, grandparents and doctors would make you think it is.

                  🕊 Leila Denmark, M.D.,
a 102-year-old pediatrician from
Alpharetta, Georgia; the oldest practicing
physician in the United States; as quoted
in
Fit Pregnancy magazine

———————————— 🍼 ————————————

NEVER EAT MORE than you can lift.

           🕊 Miss Piggy

35

I REMEMBER this very particular moment one night when I felt my first daughter move. I sat up in bed and started to cry. I woke up my husband and said, *"Oh God, someone is in here with me."* I was overwhelmed, amazed and scared. It was as though I could feel her soul.

❦ Katrine
as quoted in *Excited, Exhausted, Expecting*
by Arlene Modica Matthews

ALL THREE OF US are tied in this heart, this belly.

❦ Gladys Hindmarch, *A Birth Account*

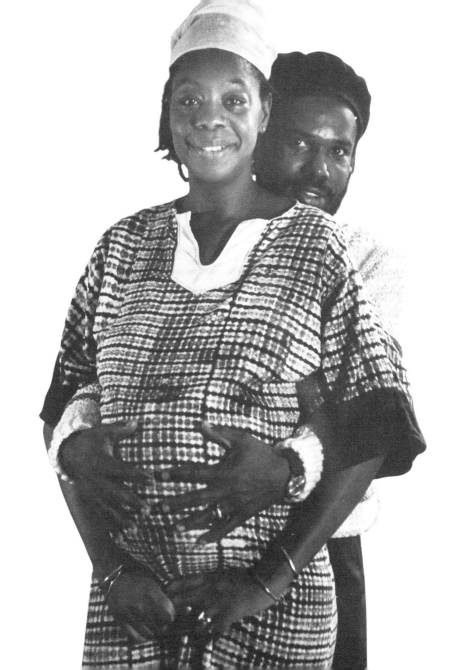

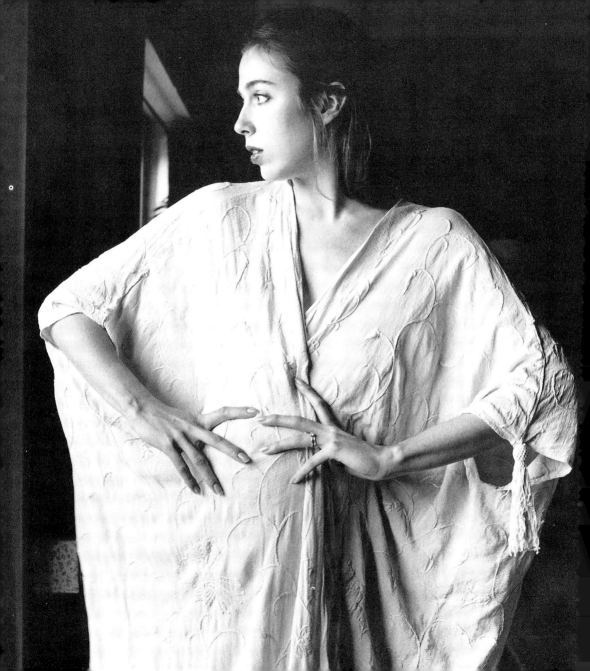

I HOLD MY BELLY, MY BABY and know I am in practice. I am the Great Mother and I am magnificent.

❧ Ann Stewart, *Womb Dance*

EVERYONE ASKS IF I AM SCARED my body will change. . . . But having a baby is what your body was meant to do. I feel like a goddess. . . . I am going to miss the way I look pregnant.

❧ Frederique van der Wal
Shape magazine

I MISS wearing belts.

❧ Kimberly Evans Rudd
The Real Deal: One Woman's Pregnancy Journal

DURING THE SECOND HALF of my pregnancy, we moved to Malibu. The beach was great. . . . I was so huge, with muscular calves from walking on the beach and swimming a lot. . . . I would sit on the deck waving, especially on the Fourth of July, so everybody on the beach was watching my progress, getting bigger and bigger until I was a beached whale.

≈ Diane Lane
as quoted on thatglow.com

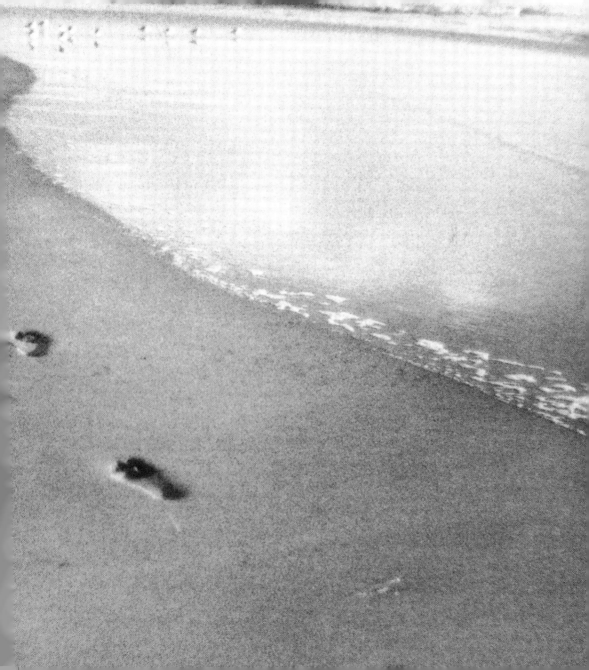

I FEEL LIKE A COW. I haven't gotten angry in weeks. I really am happy and contented. That satisfied smile must be driving some of my friends crazy with envy, or at least I hope it is.

≫ Angela Barron McBride
The Growth and Development of Mothers

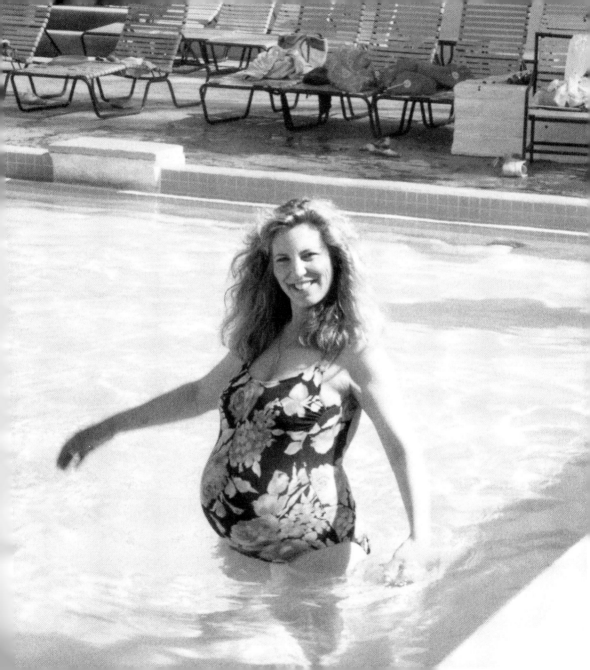

SINGING WAS A GREAT OUTLET for my emotions during pregnancy. It took the place of self-pity. So when you are in doubt, keep on singing.

≫ Deedee Bridgewater, *Birth*

I WROTE THIS STORY in part to distract myself from the daily discomforts of waiting out an overdue pregnancy (in August!). . . . I couldn't lean across my stomach to reach my desk, so I put an ironing board across the arms of a big armchair and put the computer keyboard on the ironing board.

≫ Perri Klass
as quoted in *Mothers: Twenty Stories of Contemporary Motherhood*

IN BOTH WRITING AND BIRTHING, the body, the mind, the heart are burst open wide. We open to let something greater than ourselves pass through.

≫ Gayle Brandeis, *Openings*

I DECIDED I wasn't going to be one of those women who yelled in childbirth. So when the time came, I sang ~ "The Ohio State Fight Song" ~ loud and clear. My husband told me I was off-key. I have shared this with my daughters and they have done the same.

≈ Sally Games
as quoted in *On the Birth of Your Child* by Sherry Conway Appel

---

I WAKE UP MY HUSBAND in the middle of the night to massage my legs. At least he'll be prepared for seeing to the baby in the middle of the night.

≈ Susan

TO PASS THE TIME we went to lots of movies. When we ran out of movies, we rented videos. We actually watched three videos during the early stages of labor. After the delivery, we had to ask the video store to forgive our late fee!

≈ Jennie
as quoted in *The Unofficial Guide to Having a Baby*

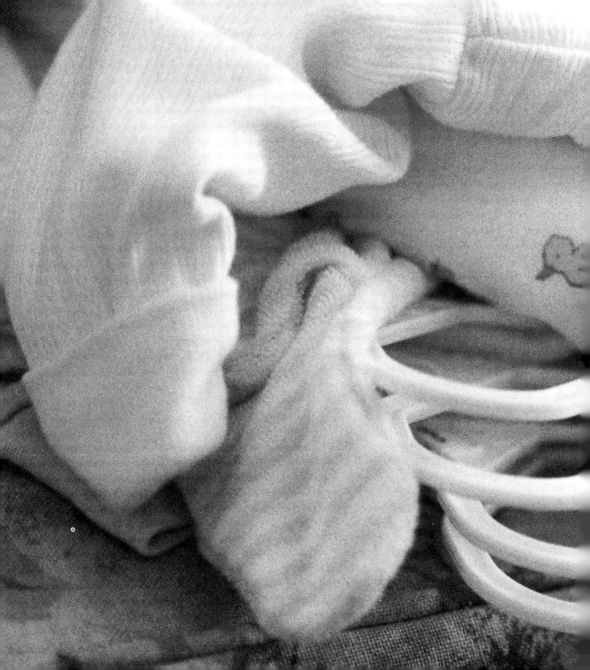

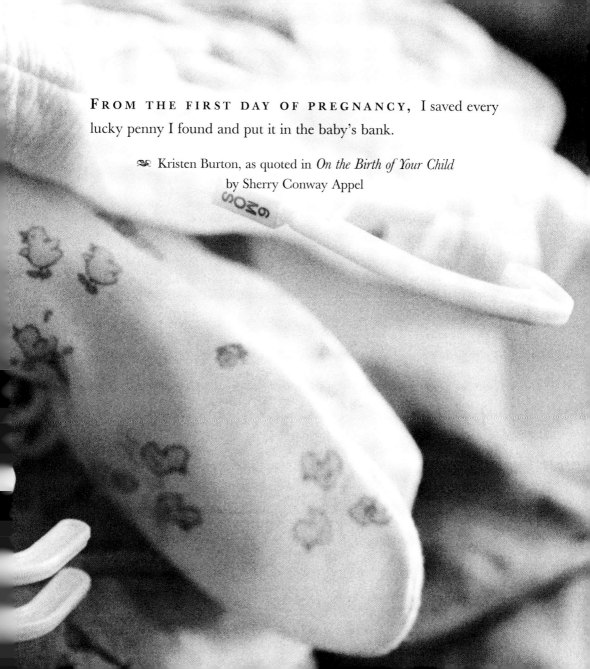

FROM THE FIRST DAY OF PREGNANCY, I saved every lucky penny I found and put it in the baby's bank.

❧ Kristen Burton, as quoted in *On the Birth of Your Child*
by Sherry Conway Appel

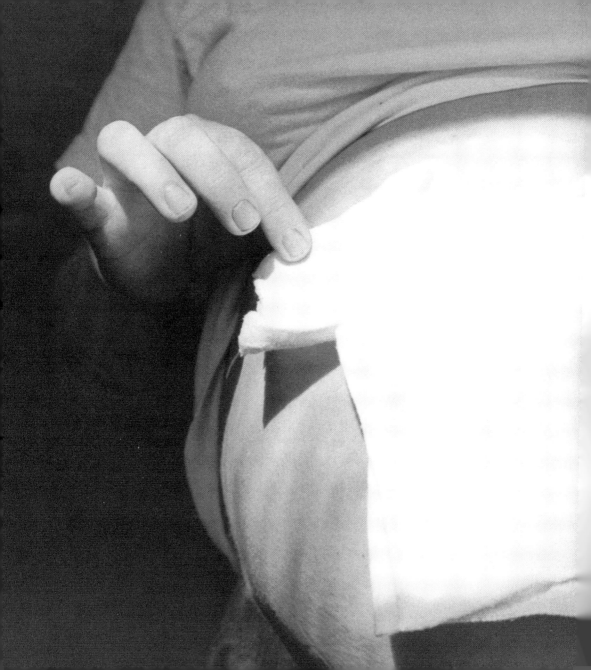

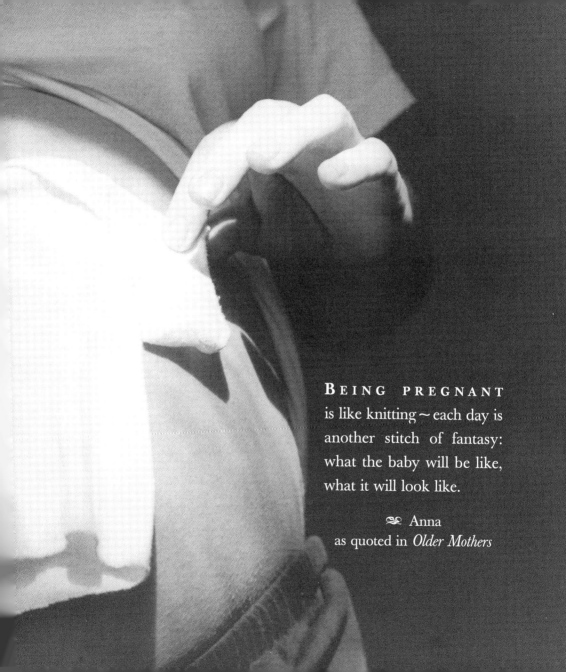

BEING PREGNANT
is like knitting ~ each day is
another stitch of fantasy:
what the baby will be like,
what it will look like.

❧ Anna
as quoted in *Older Mothers*

AS I ROLL MY CART DOWN THE AISLES, people smile at me. It isn't really me they're grinning at; it's the baby. It happens everywhere now. I always smile back because I'm the baby's link to more than just my extra weight.

≈ Bonni Goldberg, *Ants*

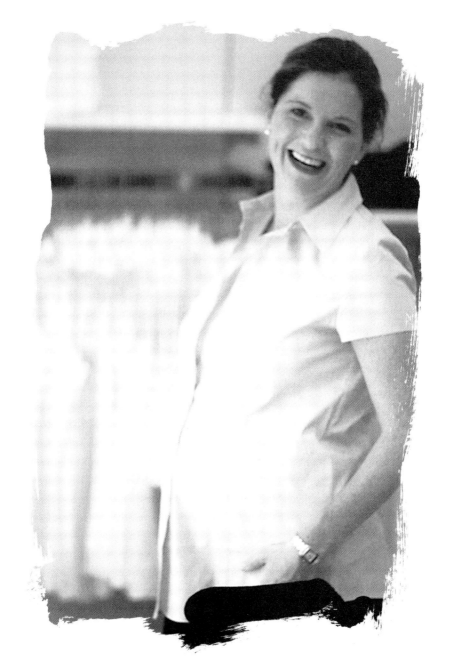

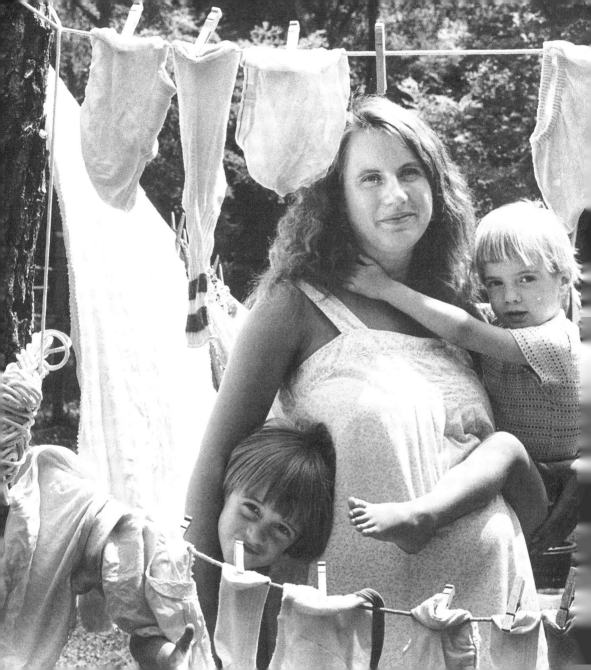

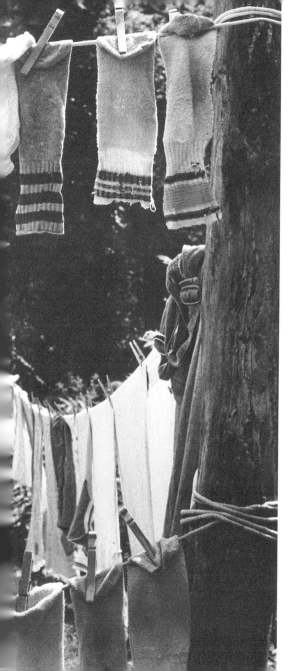

I AM NOW THIRTY-SEVEN years old and pregnant with my third child. At middle age, I am engaged in the great fight with gravity, reading up on the challenge of parenting teenagers, and juggling my OB visits amidst soccer practices and PTA meetings.

❧ Suzy Vitello
Dancing with the Paper Rose

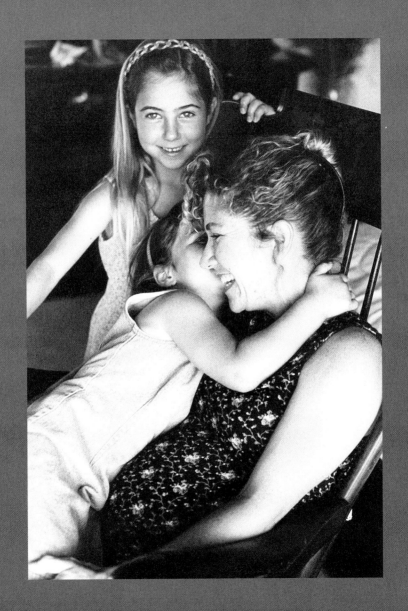

THE ACTUAL EXPERIENCE of being a mother is one of the most fulfilling I've ever had. Pregnancy was the most continuous happiness I've known.

         Gloria Vanderbilt
           Woman to Woman

THERE WERE SO MANY ADVANTAGES to being in this club. When I had little aches or pains, there seemed always to be someone to turn to who would say, "Oh yes, that happened to me." When I felt blah, sore or fat and frumpy, it helped me remember to be proud. When I felt like I was on a roller coaster ride, having given my body over to this baby, I remembered this pregnancy was earning me a badge of honor as a female.

≈ Jessie
as quoted in *Excited, Exhausted, Expecting* by Arlene Modica Matthews

I FELT LIKE I'D ENTERED this new world. It was glorious making so many deep connections with women who had maybe been somewhat reserved before. Suddenly women were confiding in me. Even my straightlaced great-aunts were telling me earthy stories.

≈ Maria
as quoted in *Excited, Exhausted, Expecting* by Arlene Modica Matthews

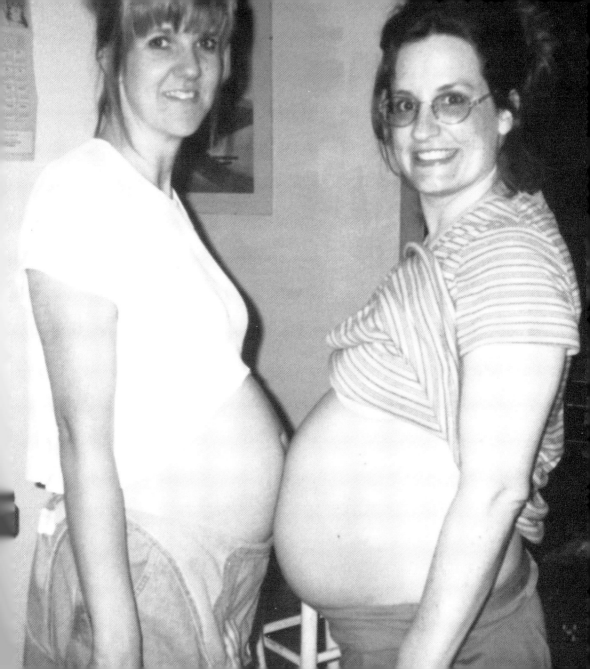

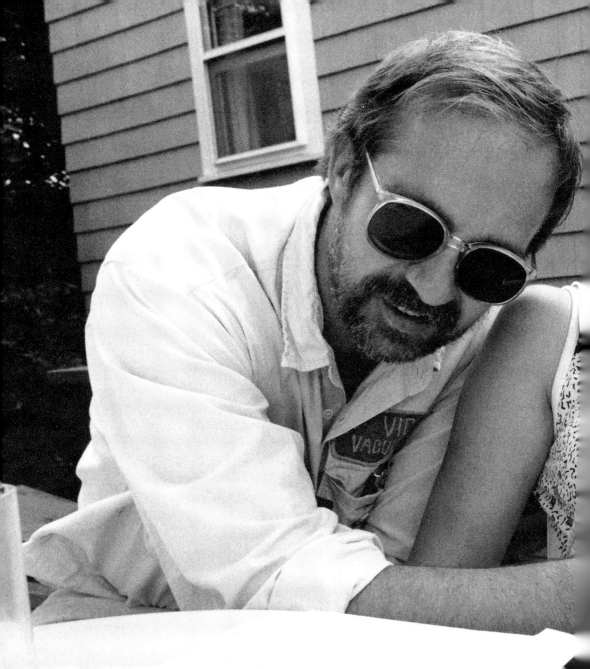

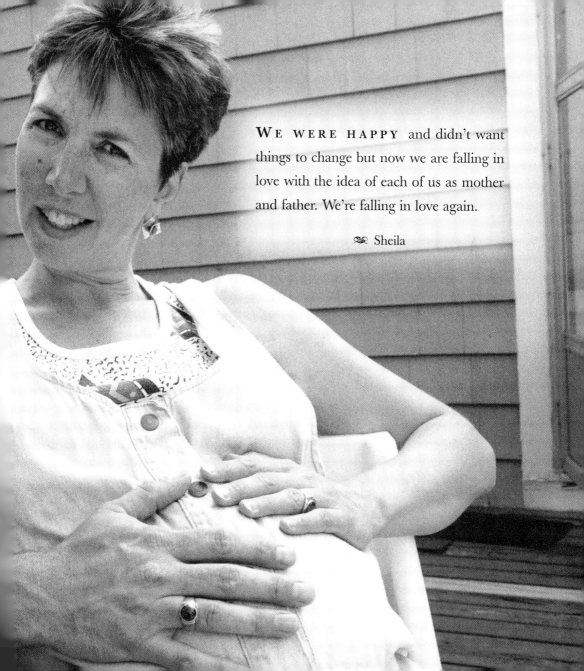

WE WERE HAPPY and didn't want things to change but now we are falling in love with the idea of each of us as mother and father. We're falling in love again.

☙ Sheila

EACH CHILD HAS ONE EXTRA LINE to your heart, which no other child can replace.

❧ Marguerite Kelly and Elia Parsons
The Mother's Almanac

I LOOKED ON CHILD REARING not only as a work of love and duty but as a profession that was fully as interesting and challenging as any honorable profession in the world and one that demanded the best that I could bring to it.

❧ Rose Kennedy

IT GOES WITHOUT SAYING that you should never have more children than you have car windows.

❧ Erma Bombeck

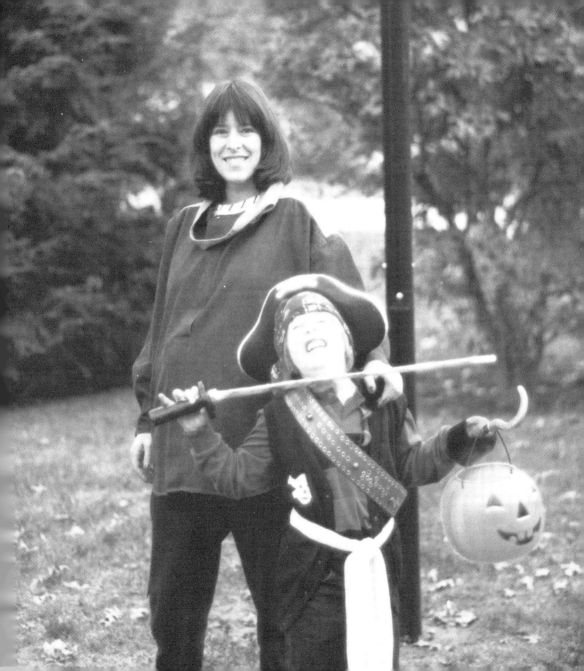

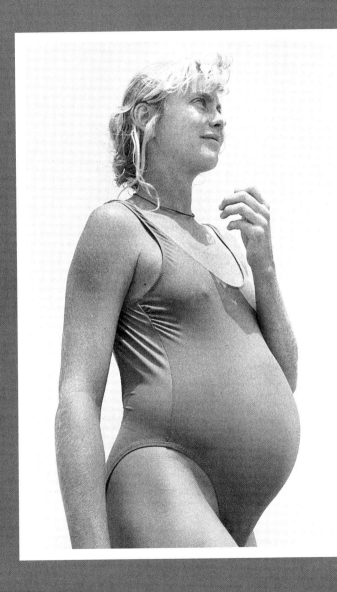

WHILE I WAS EXPECTING, I felt better than ever. I was totally connected to our baby ~ just plain exuberant!

≈ Stephanie Weiss Hubert
Shape magazine

UNLIKE THE "RADIANT GLOW" that some women had, I got edema and looked like a blow-up toy.

≈ Jo Lauria

THE NEXT EVENING we get our parents together to tell them their only children are pregnant with twins. We videotape their yahoo reaction. Life is great.

☙ Kimberly Evans Rudd
The Real Deal: One Woman's Pregnancy Journal

I DO NOT WANT to ever stop being pregnant. My body enjoys a speeded-up metabolism. My pores have closed up and my complexion is really rosy. I like to rest my hands on the jumping mound. I like to pat my stomach. I feel really arrogant and wanton.

☙ Angela Barron McBride
The Growth and Development of Mothers

THE REASON MOST PEOPLE have kids is because they get pregnant.

☙ Barbara Kingsolver
The Bean Trees

WHILE I NEVER BELIEVED the PMS insanity defense, I must confess that I can see its value for pregnant women. Between memory lapse, distorted judgment and unbearable sensitivity . . . this is not the best time to sign any binding agreement, operate heavy machinery or change your hairstyle.

⡎ Vicki Iovine
The Girlfriend's Guide to Pregnancy Daily Diary

WHEN YOU PUSH one of your tiny limbs against my belly, I am reminded what a miracle you are. . . . I will always love you.

⡎ Leah Marie Brown
as quoted in *On the Birth of Your Child*

ALL SERIOUS DARING starts from within.

⡎ Eudora Welty

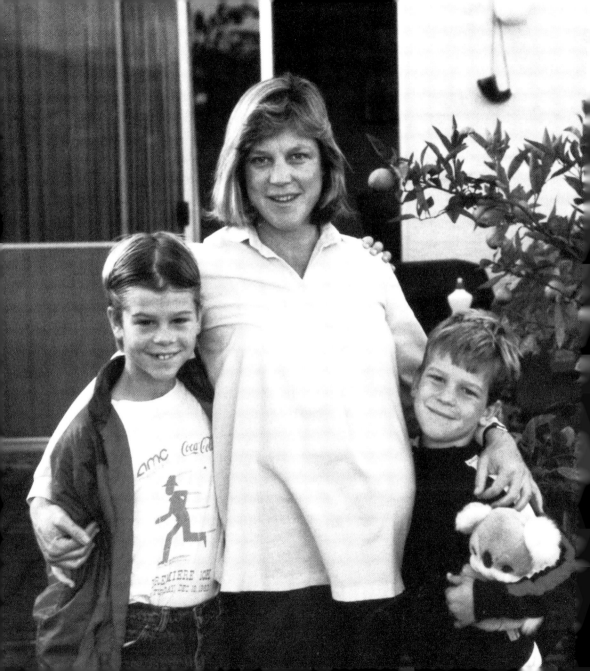

WHEN YOU ARE A MOTHER, you are never really alone in your thoughts. You are connected to your child and to all those who touch your lives. A mother always has to think twice, once for herself and once for her child.

 Sophia Loren

SUDDENLY, I AM LESS JUDGMENTAL of my friends who have kids. I don't blame them for their kids' obnoxious behavior in the hope they won't blame me for mine.

 Dolores

YOU WERE SUCH A WANTED BABY. I would rub my belly in awe of your growing. Sit motionless waiting for your kicks and stretches. Think of you, wonder about you, wait for you ~ totally caught in the miracle of your coming to life. First child, child of hope, child of commitment.

❧ Julie Owen Edwards

BEING PREGNANT, as it turns out, is not about keeping in, but instead, it is the first step in letting go. Allowing a part of myself to cleave into something completely its own, and having the grace to attend this miracle of life while respecting the whole person that I continue to be.

❧ Suzy Vitello
Dancing with the Paper Rose

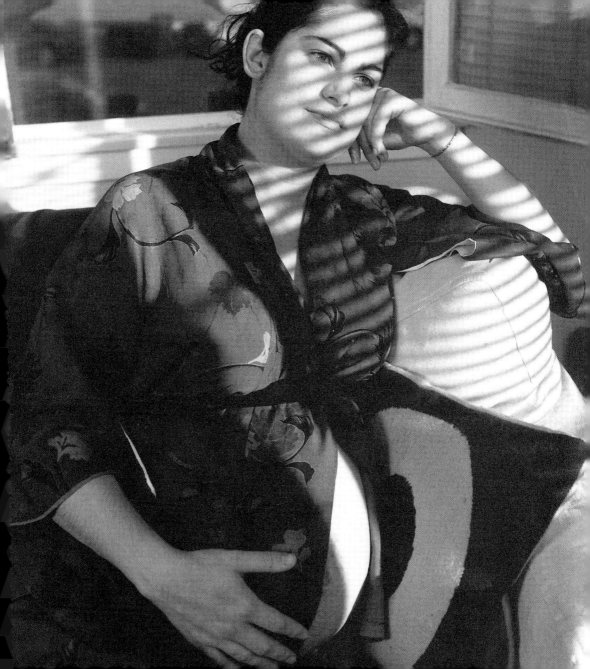

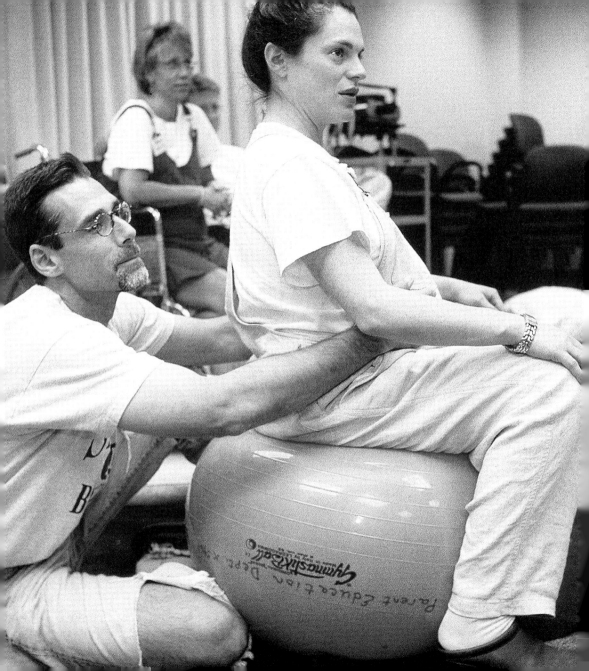

THIS BABY IS MY MASTERPIECE, my creation, my work of art. Our child will be the proof of the love my husband and I have for each other.

> ❧ Angela Barron McBride
> *The Growth and Development of Mothers*

THERE'S A LOT MORE to being a woman than being a mother, but there's a hell of a lot more to being a mother than most people suspect.

> ❧ Roseanne

IS IT WORTH ALL OF THIS just to get presents on Mother's Day?

> ❧ Nancy

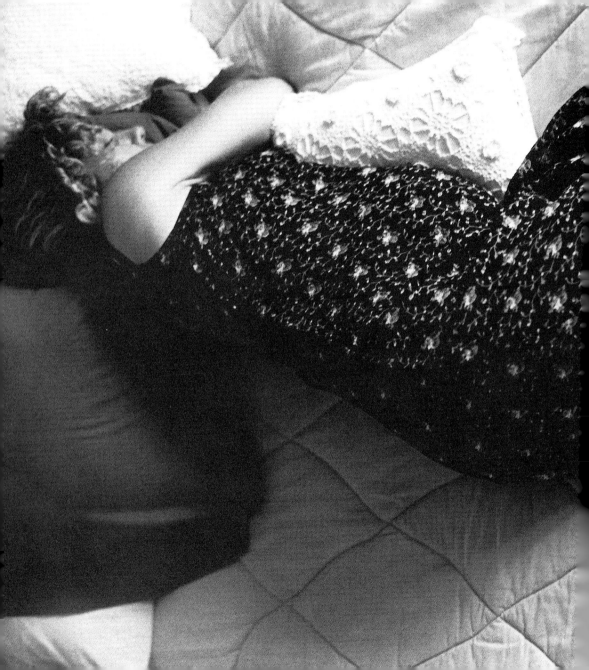

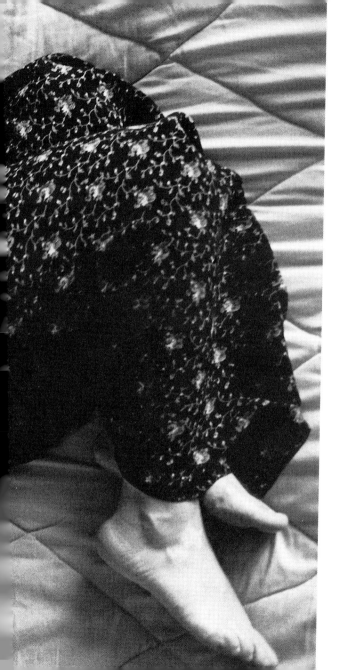

NOW I WAS someone who ate like a wolf, napped like a cat and dreamed like a madwoman.

≈ Marni Jackson
The Mother Zone

I LOVE ROCKING CHAIRS. Every night after work I collapse into one and fall into a state of arrested animation. My body becomes completely still except perhaps for my toe, pushing and rocking, and my mind calms. I picture myself clasping my baby to my heart on the rocking chair, rocking away with her into a land of dreams and beyond. My baby!

❧ Dawn M. Tucksmith
Secrets and Dreams

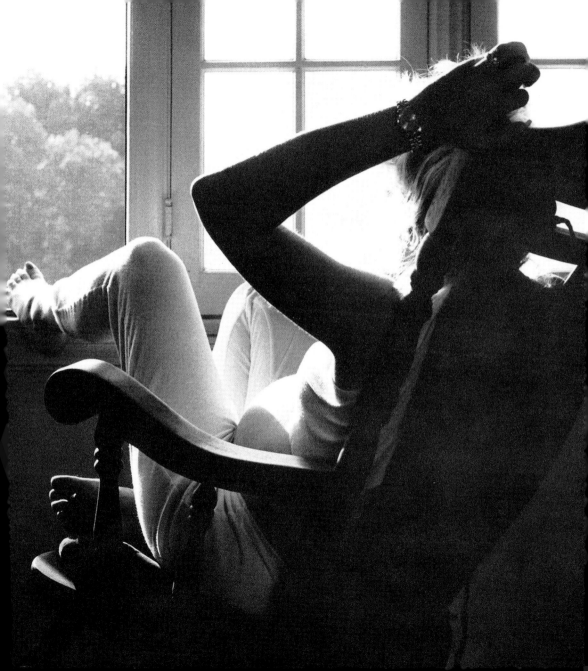

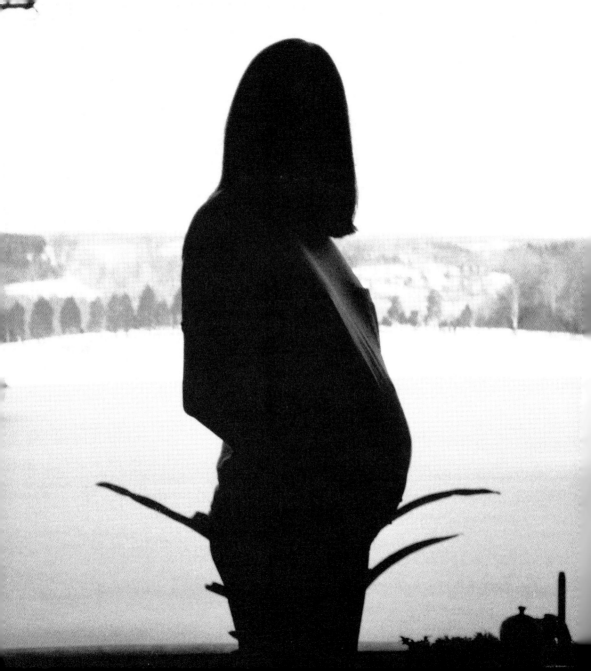

EVEN MY SHADOW IS PREGNANT, I noticed one Saturday. I was nearing the end of my second trimester. My stomach was big and hard and lopsided, and strangers always looked at it before meeting my eyes.

༄ Carol Weston
From Here to Maternity

WE'RE PREGNANT! And to think we complained about some of the cheap hotels on the road. I guess those lumpy beds aren't so bad after all!

❧ Kimberly Evans Rudd

The Real Deal: One Woman's Pregnancy Journal

IT SOMETIMES HAPPENS, even in the best families, that a baby is born. This is not necessarily a cause for alarm. The important thing is to keep your wits about you and borrow some money.

❧ Elinor Goulding Smith

The Complete Book of Absolutely Perfect Baby and Child Care

SUCH SOLICITOUS CARE I have never had. Chairs pulled out for me, things picked up for me, milk offered me, an arm offered for high steps. . . . At first it bothered me; now I think it rather a relief ~ sometimes very funny and sometimes nice.

        ❧ Anne Morrow Lindbergh

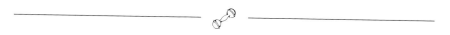

THE TROUBLE with getting introspective when you're pregnant is that you never know who you might run into.

        ❧ Carrie Fisher
        Delusions of Grandma

WE WENT OUT to a big family dinner. How wonderful not to feel that you have to offer to wash the dishes.

        ❧ Angela Barron McBride
        The Growth and Development of Mothers

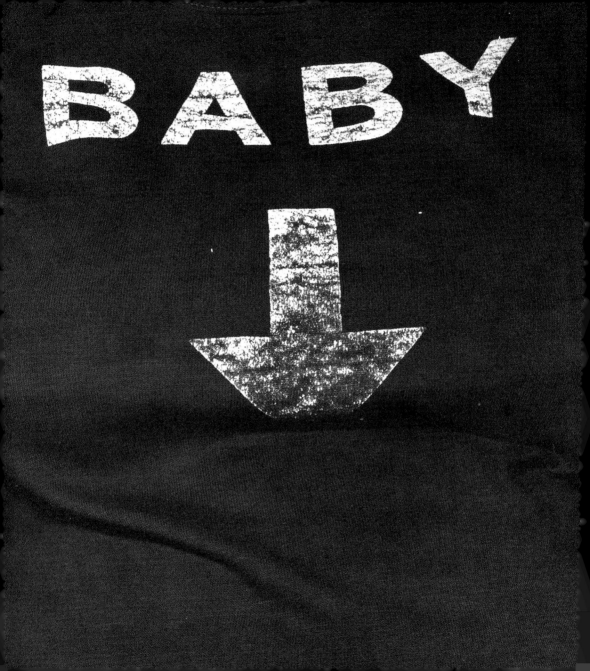

MY 2½-YEAR-OLD NIECE hugged and kissed my growing belly while telling me that she loved my tummy ache.

꙳ Rosalie Deguzman
Shape magazine

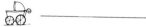

WHAT IS GOOD FOR MORNING SICKNESS?

Candice Bergen: Nothing.

Kelly Preston: Vitamin K (if deficient), saltines, eating small meals continuously, bananas, potassium tablets. I also chewed on ginger (crystallized tastes like candy) and that was really helpful.

Marie Osmond: Setting the alarm for noon.

꙳ as quoted on thatglow.com

YOU ARE ENTIRELY ENGROSSED in your own body and the life it holds. It is as if you were in the grip of a powerful force; as if a wave had lifted you above and beyond everyone else. In this way there is always a part of a pregnant woman that is unreachable and is reserved for the future.

꿈 Sophia Loren
Mother's Nature

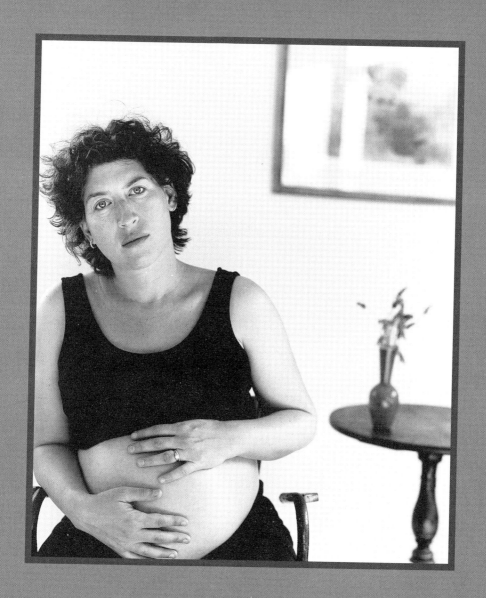

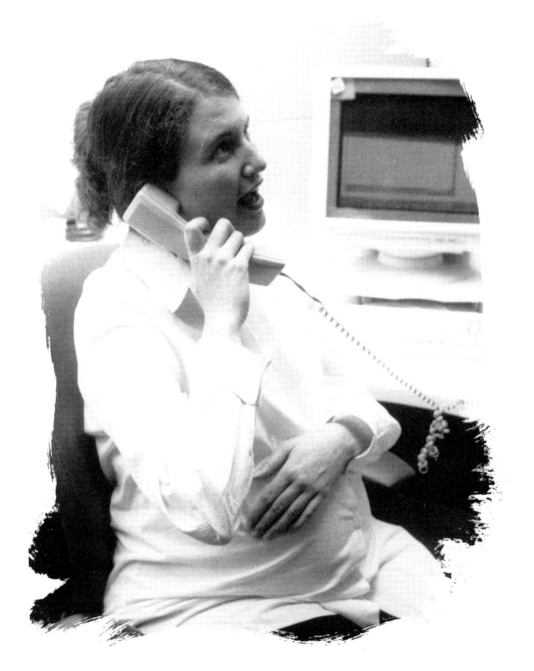

I WAS SITTING AT MY DESK transcribing some notes when I felt a strange flutter. My baby began, ever so gently, to soft-shoe his way across my abdomen.

᪢ Arlene Modica Matthews
Excited, Exhausted, Expecting

ANY MOTHER COULD PERFORM THE JOBS of several air-traffic controllers with ease.

᪢ Lisa Alther

IF PREGNANCY WERE A BOOK, they would cut the last two chapters.

≈ Nora Ephron
Heartburn

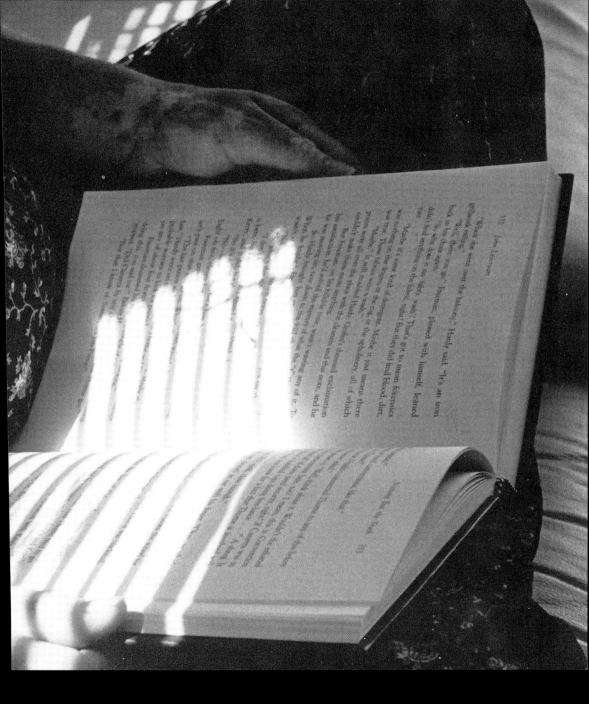

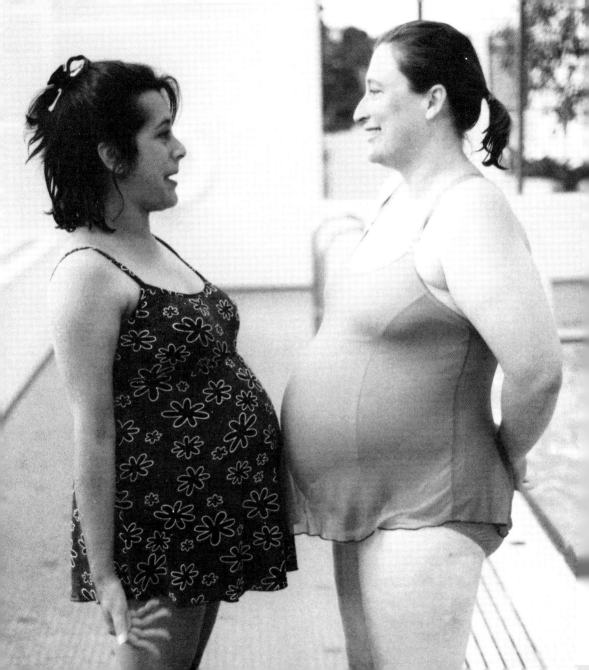

I WAS SLOWLY taking on the dimensions of a chest of drawers.

❧ Maria Augusta Trapp
The Story of the Trapp Family Singers

LIKE THE WEDDING DRESS, the maternity dress attempts to make the woman a package, complete with ribbons and bows, as if to be handed to whoever owns her.

 Christine Pakkala
as quoted on salon.com

I JUST HAUL OUT something stretchy and hope it fits. And if it doesn't, I find something else and hope it stretches.

 Jada Pinkett Smith
as quoted on thatglow.com

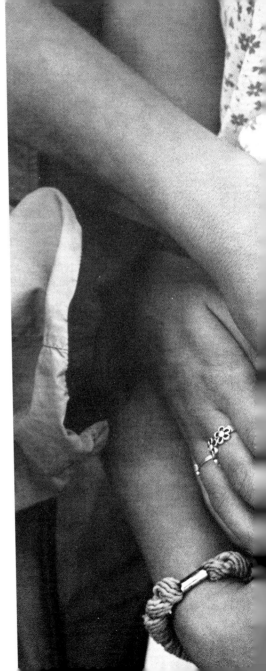

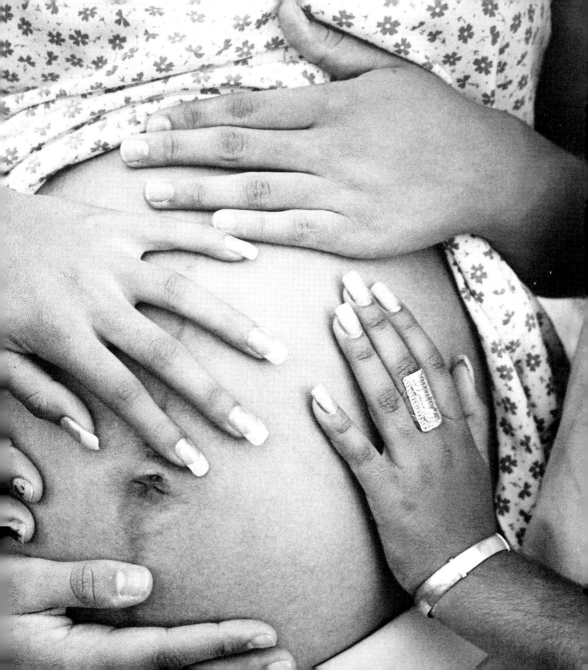

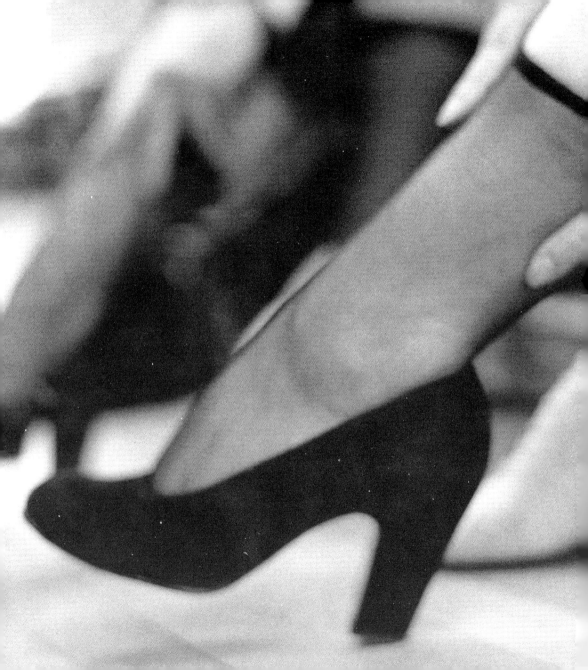

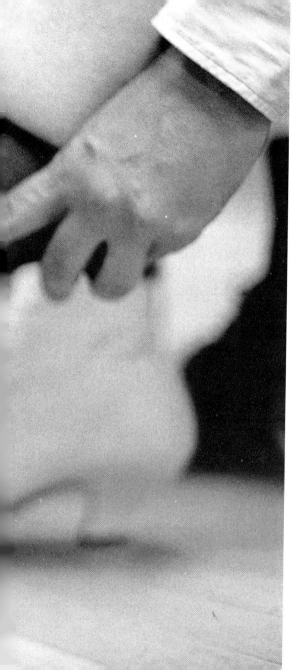

DID YOU BUY anything for yourself during your pregnancy that you consider a real indulgence?

Rosanna Arquette: Shoes! My foot grew half an inch so I had to restock my fancy ones.

❧ as quoted on thatglow.com

MY **BABY WILL** know a mother figure who sings out loud, takes long walks on the beach with him at daybreak, and lies down on the floor surrounded by our animals, plants and the love of a man as interested in spirit as I am.

℮ Ellen R. Klein
Birth of a Woman

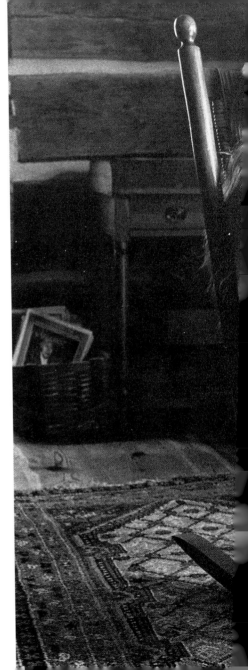

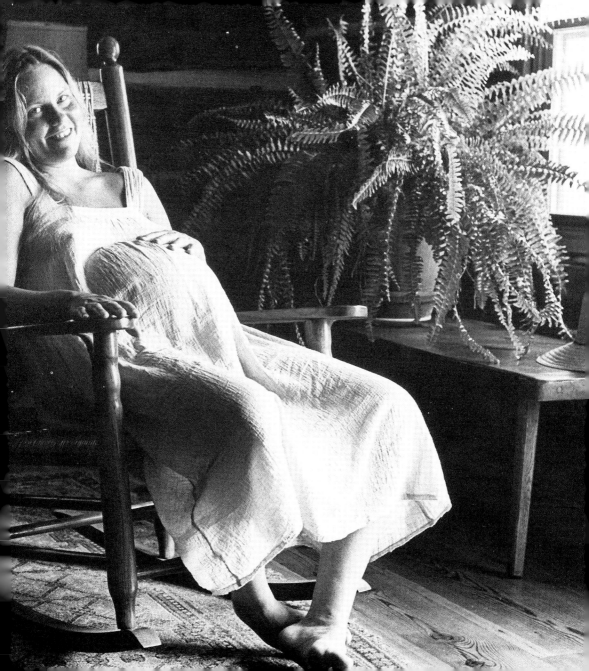

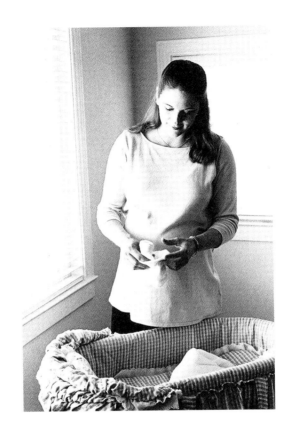

NOURISH BEGINNINGS, let us nourish beginnings. . . .

≈ Muriel Rukeyser
"Elegy in Joy," *The Green Wave*

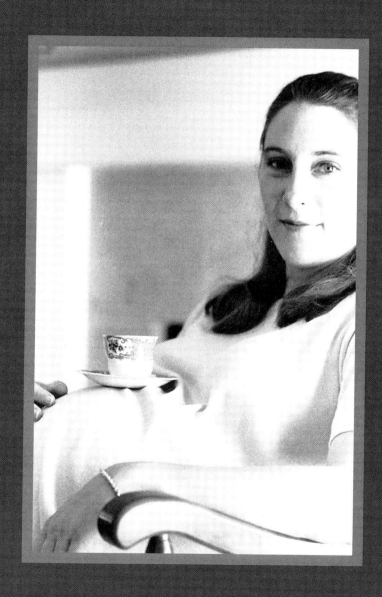

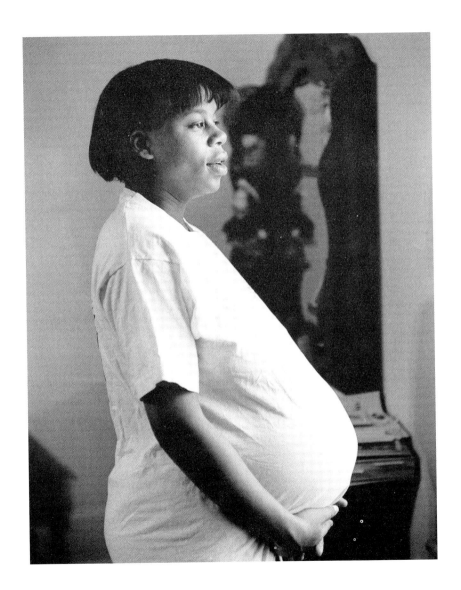

IF YOU ARE PREGNANT, you are in the midst of a rich, mysterious and enlightening period of your life; an odyssey and metamorphosis all in one.

≈ Bonni Goldberg
The Spirit of Pregnancy

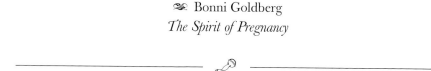

THAT IS WHAT LEARNING IS. You suddenly understand something you've understood your whole life, but in a new way.

≈ Doris Lessing

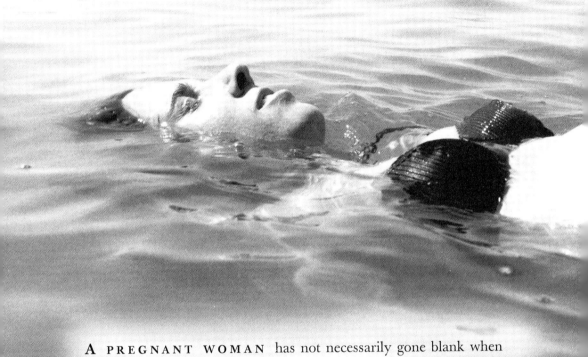

A PREGNANT WOMAN has not necessarily gone blank when she falls silent or lets herself float along in a foggy mood. She is, so to speak, sitting next to the flow of life, close to its source.

❧ Arthur and Libby Coleman
Pregnancy: The Psychological Experience

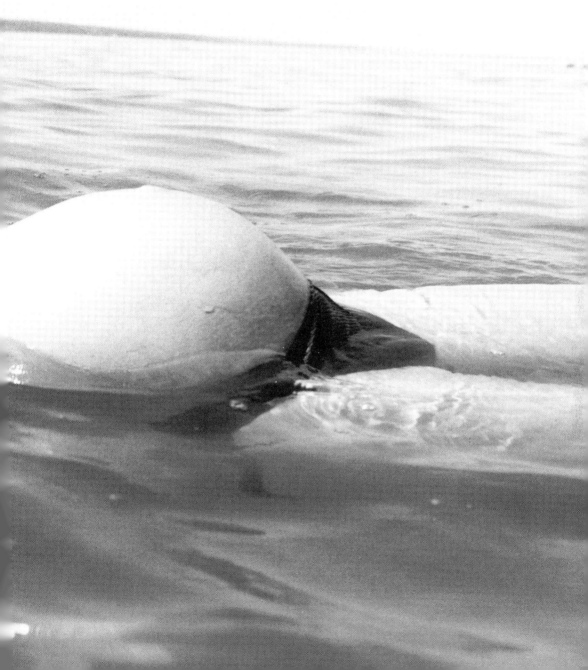

DURING THE CALM, ROTUND FINAL MONTHS of my first pregnancy, I wanted to meet the little person who would be my daughter, but I also wanted to relish the mystery ~ and anxiety ~ of not knowing. As long as my child was inside me, I knew where she was and had a sense from her pokes and prods and hiccups of how she was, even if I didn't yet know who she was. Pregnancy seemed to be one of the most satisfying stories, deeply suspenseful and hinting at every step of its own magnificent resolution. And when the pleasure of suspense threatened to deteriorate into worry, all I'd have to do was give a nudge or eat some penne, and my little mystery would start bouncing around, assuring me that she was fine.

೪ Joanna Scott
as quoted on salon.com

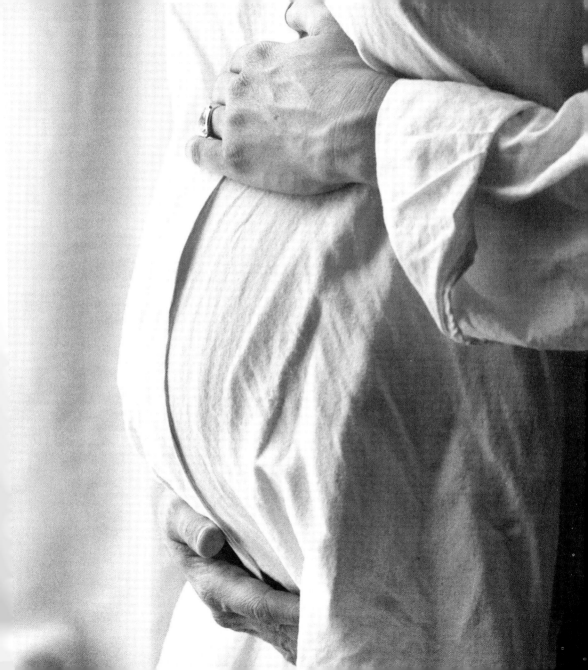

EVERY MORNING on the instant you wake up, you see a huge, blown-up version of the baby in your mind's eye. You remain absolutely still, so as not to ignite the heaving mechanism, and dwell instead on the waving hands, the shimmering dark and light image that flickers like a movie from the 1920s.

❧ Anna Purves, *Seen and Not Seen*

THE DEDICATED LIFE is the life worth living. You must give with your whole heart.

❧ Annie Dillard

I HAVE ACCEPTED FEAR as a part of life, specifically the fear of change. . . I have gone ahead despite the pounding in the heart that says: turn back. . . .

❧ Erica Jong

AND IN THAT INSTANT, the baby kicked, not fluttered, but kicked, kicked hard. "I'm getting out of here one day," the feet pounded.

> ❧ Joan Connor
> *The Age of Discovery*

I FEEL LIKE A MAN BUILDING A BOAT in his basement which he may not be able to get out through the door. Trapped, frantic and trapped.

> ❧ Abigail Lewis
> *An Interesting Condition*

TO LOVE IS TO RECEIVE a glimpse of heaven.

> ❧ Karen Sunde

ABOUT A WEEK BEFORE MY SON was born, a peace and calm came over me and I actually looked forward to experiencing the power and beauty of giving birth. Perhaps that was my hormones kicking in, in preparation for the coming birth. And I did have a wonderful birth experience ~ one where I was in control and not panicky or upset.

≈ Tracy
as quoted in *The Unofficial Guide to Having a Baby*
by Ann Douglas and John Sussman

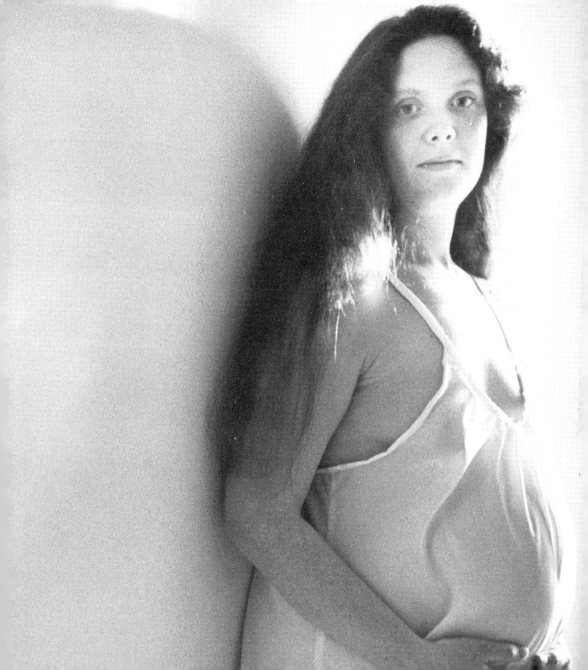

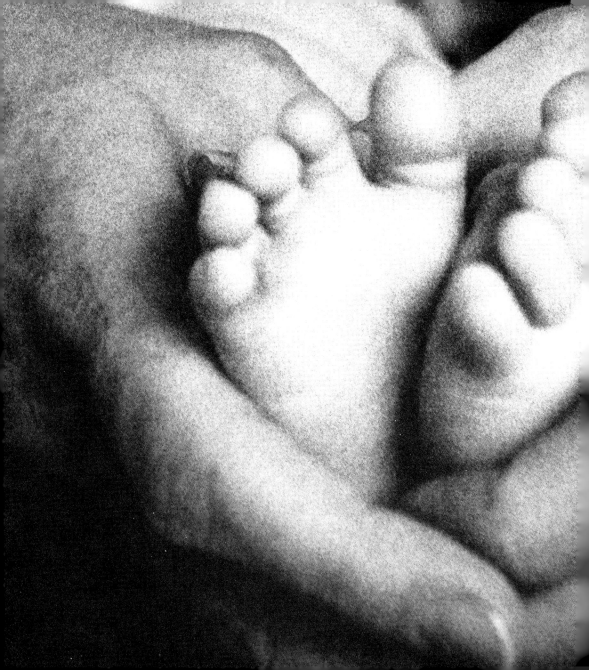

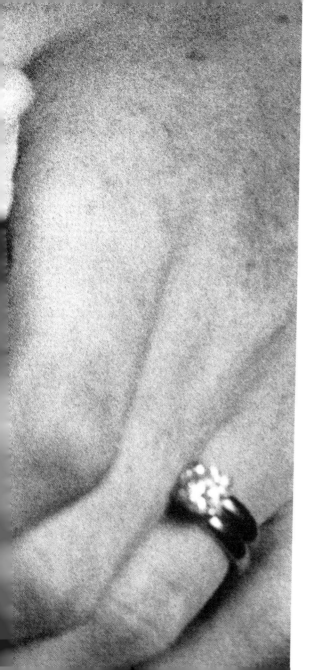

GIVING BIRTH is life's
most powerful realization of
a miracle.

≈ Catherine Milinaire
Birth

ACKNOWLEDGMENTS

THE WORDS

The quotes used in this book were culled from many, many sources, but there's one book I especially want to acknowledge. I discovered *The Spirit of Pregnancy* by Bonni Goldberg (Contemporary Books, 2000) early in my research, and what a find it was! Here is an utterly brilliant and enchanting collection of stories, poems and essays about pregnancy. Each one is a little marvel. I highly recommend Goldberg's book to anyone interested in pregnancy, maternity, babies or how women think about themselves.

THE PICTURES

The art in this book represents an eclectic mixture of art photography and family snapshots. In pulling this book together, I called upon my friends and family. Fortunately for me, many of my dearest friends are talented photographers who amazed me with their own work and suggested other photographers to the project. Others were extremely generous about sharing their snapshots. I am grateful to all of them for their contributions. I also want to thank my very dear friend Ella Stewart, and Pat Tan and John Smallwood.

≈ Linda Sunshine

CREDITS

Mayra Barba, 90

Susan Dorenter, 5, 61

Richard Glenn, 43

Mark Goodman, 80

Dede Hatch, 2, 26, 29, 34, 46, 48, 58, 100, 103

Marsha Heckman, 6, 21, 22, 51, 84, 88, 96, 97

Mary Motley Kalergis, 24, 37, 52, 62, 94, 98, 106

Dolores Lusitana, 1, 30, 40, 54, 72, 86, 92, 108

Margaretta Mitchell, 33, 38

Judy Montague, 14, 57, 66, 112

Keri Pickett, 10, 16, 70

Allyn Rosensweig, 75

Jessica Shokrian, 69, 83

Scott Thode, 19

Clark Wakabayashi, 12, 76

Laura Ross White, 20

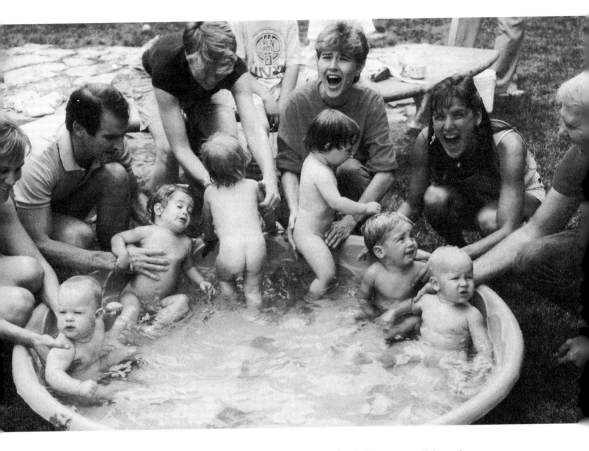

All the adults around the pool are siblings. The babies were all born between February and September of 1985 and are first cousins.

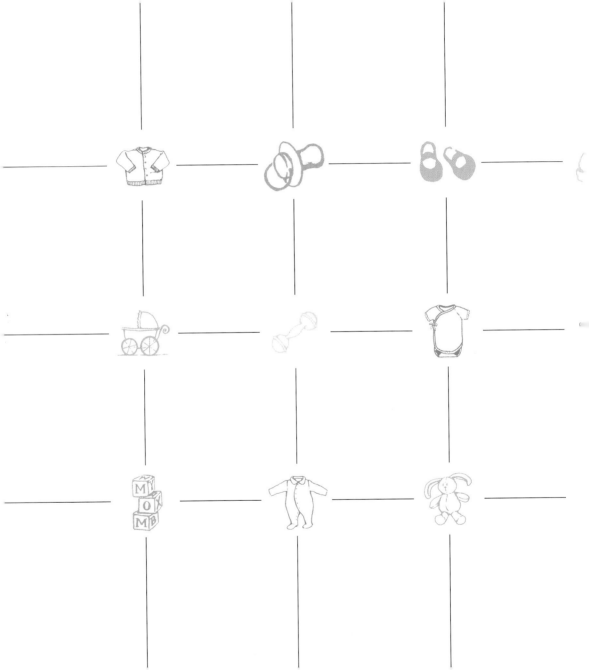